Couch to Career

Becoming a Nurse

D1002549

JETEIA L. BENSON RN,
MSN,FNP-C

ISBN: 0-9982482-1-5
ISBN-13: 978-0-9982482-1-9

DEDICATION

This book was written to help you reach your dream of becoming a nurse. May it help propel you from your couch to an exciting new career in nursing.

To my Nana Dolores and Pops Grady who got to witness me accomplish major goals while being my motivational support system, but did not get to witness the release of this book. This one's for you. I am so glad I could make you proud!

CONTENTS

ACKNOWLEDGMENTS

I can not acknowledge anyone until I take time for thanking God for filling me with the courage and determination to put this information out in the world. Next, I want to thank my two biggest cheerleaders my mother and David my love. Finally, I would like to thank my book editor Michele A. Bararad of Urban Book Editor LLC., for guiding me through this process. I would also like to thank Heather Hargrow Designs for my cover designs.

1 INTRODUCTION

I would like to introduce myself. Hello, my name is Jeteia, and I am a nurse. I decided to write this book as a guide for all those who feel like I once did, lost with no career direction. If you are reading this, you are likely interested in becoming a nurse. Let me pause and say nurses are awesome! Now, I'll get back to my story.

I was about five years old when I told my mother I wanted to be a "baby doctor." That was right around the time my little brother was born. I helped my mother as much as possible with the baby. Helping with my brother lit a fire in my soul, and I decided I wanted to pursue a career in healthcare. Fast forward, I worked hard throughout high-school and was able to go to the college of my choice. I chose Fisk University in Nashville, Tennessee. I excelled in college, majoring in Biology with the goal of going to medical school. It was not until after graduation that I realized I no longer wanted to pursue that goal.

In my opinion, I had done the worst possible thing; I had graduated from college with no direction. I decided to attend graduate school for public health, but Hurricane Katrina had other plans for me. I landed back at home still with no direction. I then began to pray. I prayed hard. I prayed day in and day out. I prayed tirelessly. I prayed consistently.

One day, I wandered into a beauty supply store and ran into another Fiskite. She shared with me that she had felt like I did. After graduation, she had no career direction either. She was recently accepted into a nursing program and had fallen in love. After our talk, I researched nursing, but I was not convinced right away. The more I researched, the more I saw all the wonderful things nurses do. I remembered all the kind, dedicated nurses I had encountered throughout my life. But what really sealed the deal was the flexibility in nursing. There are literally dozens of paths for nurses. I could be a floor nurse, a research nurse, a nurse that runs clinical trials, a legal nurse, and the list goes on. I was sold! Nursing was the field for me.

In November 2007, I decided to apply for the program my Fisk sister told me about. I did not bother looking for other programs. I was accepted and set to start an accelerated nursing program the following January. The program was a year and a half and the time whizzed by so fast I can hardly remember it.

I said all that to say if you have ever felt lost with no direction, hopeless, unsure, and/or unclear on your career path this is the PERFECT BOOK FOR YOU! This book will guide you from your couch to a fabulous career in nursing. There will be a step by step guide including all the important need-to-know details about how to become a nurse. Stay tuned.

2 ARE YOU READY?

You are reading this because you have decided or need to be convinced that Nursing is the career for you. What is a nurse? The definition of a nurse is one who is trained to care for the sick or injured. That is the official definition, but a nurse is a lot more than that. Nurses are the primary caregivers in the hospital. They are at the bedside with patients 24 hours a day. The nurse carries out the physicians' orders. Nurses monitor and assess patients and perform interventions to get the patient well enough to be discharged. The nurse is also responsible for educating the patient about preventing further illness, appropriate self-care, and specific discharge instructions. Nurses are the educators of the medical field.

Nurses can wear many hats. Here are examples of different types of nurses: Pediatric nurses, critical care nurses, cardiac nurses, dialysis nurses, medical surgical nurses, orthopedic nurses, labor and delivery nurses, neonatal intensive care nurses, diabetes educator nurses, critical care transport nurses, telephone triage nurses, informatics nurses, and nurse administrators, nurse practitioners, nurse midwives, nursing instructors, clinical nurse educators, home care nurses, and legal nurses just to name a few.

Now, I want you to make a list of reasons why you think nursing is a good fit for you, better yet, why you are a good fit for nursing. Now let's take a long hard look at the list. If your list includes making a ton of money you may want to think about this more. I am not judging you because this is true that in some cases you can make a ton of money, but I do not think that is good enough reason to go into nursing. If you ask any nurse, they would say doing it for the money is not going to help you make it through those long day shifts and even longer night shifts.

I took a quick poll of nurses I know, and everyone had a different reason that inspired them to go into the field. Still, the common denominator was people. We all wanted to help people. Nursing is one of the most selfless careers on the planet. Whatever your reason be, make sure it is so deeply rooted that you can revert back to it at times you are questioning the journey or your decision. Evaluate your reason before moving on.

After you have reflected on your reasoning, always remember, you have what it takes, so do what it takes! Develop a positive mindset now. See yourself as a Nurse before you start. Failure is not an option. Do not allow you to talk yourself out of this. What are you waiting for? STOP making excuses. If you know you would make an amazing nurse, keep reading. If you do not think you would make an amazing nurse, keep reading.

3 DETERMINATION

There is no way this guide could be written without acknowledging the creator for allowing us to become successful. You may not believe in God. That matters not. The point is, whatever support system you need to gather, do so. You have to believe in yourself enough to accomplish any goal you set your mind to.

Repeat this mantra after me: I ROCK, AND I WILL BE AN AWESOME NURSE!

The key to your success will be to begin building your confidence before you get into nursing. Think about your reasons for wanting to become a nurse. Whatever those reasons are, know you can do it. You have power and authority over every situation. Pursuing a career in nursing is a big decision and an even bigger commitment. Believe that no task is too big for you. You definitely can do it. Always empower yourself. The definition of empower is to give authority, to enable, to permit. By definition, you need to grant yourself permission to succeed. Give yourself the authority to set goals and stick to them. Set the goals up and knock them down one by one.

Personality self-check: Are you determined? Resilient? Motivated?

You will need all of these characteristics to make it through the steps in this guide. Determination means having a firmness of purpose or the process of establishing something exactly. The definition of resilience is; the capacity to recover quickly or toughness. And motivated means stimulated interest in or enthusiasm for doing something. Are you tough and enthusiastic about becoming a nurse? Think about it because you should be.

Result is a verb meaning to spring, arise, or proceed as a consequence of actions. It also is a noun, something that happens as a consequence; outcome. What results are you trying to get? What is your outcome? What is at stake for you? You need to be determined to accomplish your goals, resilient in taking the necessary steps, and remain motivated throughout the process. Remember why you are doing this. Keep the end goal in mind.

4 BABY STEPS

Have you ever considered becoming a nursing assistant? I truly believe ALL nurses should start out as nursing assistants. This is not required; however, doing so will give you insight into nurses' duties and responsibilities. Working as a nursing assistant also will encourage you to get "down and dirty" in nursing. What I mean by that is as a nursing assistant you are primarily the patient's assistant. You will be responsible for many activities of daily living in addition to being an extra set of eyes for the nurse. You cannot be a good leader if you are not able to follow.

Becoming a nursing assistant is not a national standard requirement, however, over the last several years an increasing number of nursing programs are adding that criterion. Programs want to produce quality, well-rounded nurses. The goal is to produce nurses that companies are begging to hire. Will you be one of them?

FACT: Many nursing programs do not require you to be a nursing assistant, but truth is, they may consider those who were over someone who was not. You want to increase your chances of being hired.

What exactly is a nursing assistant?

A Certified Nursing Assistant, or CNA, helps patients or clients with healthcare needs under the supervision of a Registered Nurse (RN) or a Licensed Practical Nurse (LPN). The term is used interchangeably with Nursing Assistant (NA), a Patient Care Assistant (PCA), or a State Tested Nurse Aid (STNA). This is a great first step to getting into the field of nursing. You need to possess a lot of the same qualities a nurse needs to have with regard to the patient population. There are thousands of CNA or STNA programs available. The list spans from private programs to long-term care facility programs, to some colleges that offer programs.

There are several programs available that will fit your needs. The best part is that you can almost tailor the program to fit your scheduling needs; there are weekend only options, evening options, or week-day options. Figure out which is going to work for you. Most programs are affordable or offer students payment plans. There are also some long-term care facilities that will train you in exchange for you working at their facility. Nursing assistant programs tend to be short, lasting between one and three weeks in length. A good place to start the search for CNA schools is www.allnuringschools.com. Another website that has good resources and information for CNAs is www.nursingassistants.net. Some programs will require a high-school diploma for enrollment; others will not. Whatever your need is, you should be able to find an appropriate program.

After the completion of a training program, the nursing assistant sits for a state administered test to become certified. The exam is done in two parts: a written portion and a clinical portion. The written test is usually not too difficult. The website www.nursingassistants.net offers sample questions for you to practice for the examination. The clinical part is a bit harder. You have to bring a friend with you in order to complete this portion. The friend will serve as your patient on whom you demonstrate your skills to the examiner. When you achieve this certification, you can proceed with your job search.

FACT: The job outlook is positive! Wages vary from state to state but the national average hourly pay for a Nursing Assistant is anywhere between $8.55 to $16.62. Source: www.mycnajobs.com/caregiver-cna-pay/

According to the BLS, the top 10 percent of nursing assistants earned more than $36,170.

Nursing Career	Median Annual Salary
Licensed Practical and Licensed Vocational Nurse	$42,490
Registered Nurses	$66,640
Medical Assistants	$29,960
Physical Therapist Assistants and Aides	$41,640

Resource: www.allnursingschools.com

Now that you have become a nursing assistant, I advise you to look for a job in an area that interests you. For example, if you are interested in working with children, look into getting a job at a facility that cares for pediatrics. That way you will have an idea about the inner-workings before you finish nursing school. If you are not able to get a job in your dream area, do not sweat it. Any experience is good experience.

5 NURSING PROGRAMS

This chapter will provide a brief overview of the types of nursing programs available. Please do your research before you enroll in any program. My advice to you would be to become a member of different groups or online communities of students to get the real low down information on the nursing schools. Programs come in all shapes and sizes, and no one size fits all. Look for a program that can be worked into your life, not something you have to completely alter your life to attend.

There are several things to consider when searching for a nursing school. Please take the time to look into the following criteria before enrolling in a particular program.

1.   Location of the school. Is the school easily accessible to you? Will

you be able to commute or live on campus?

2.   What is the specialty of the school? For example, there are some schools that only offer 2-year nursing programs and some that offer both two and four-year programs.

3.   Is the size of the school important to you? Will there be very large classes or smaller, more intimate classes?

4.   Is the school accredited? This means the school is officially recognized for meeting specific requirements of academic excellence. Jobs like to make sure you attended an accredited school so they know the quality of nurse they are hiring and that you received a good nursing education. This also means the program takes your education seriously enough to follow the standards set by the accrediting bodies in the field and have met all

the specific criteria to educate and produce quality nurses.

It is also a good idea to look at the schools National Council Licensure Examination (NCLEX) pass rate. This gives an indication of how well prepared the students are who have gone through the program. Lastly, you must consider the tuition costs. What is it going to cost you to attend nursing school? Is that feasible for you? There are often financial aid options available for those who qualify. Be sure you have found out as much about the program as possible before you apply.

6 GETTING INTO NURSING SCHOOL

Nursing schools usually have their own required or suggested prerequisites for eligibility for the nursing entrance exam of their choice. Some require that you complete certain coursework or pass other exams. Often, you must have earned at least a certain grade point average in order to register for the test. There are also suggestions for timing the test so that you will be able to achieve competitive results. There are several nursing school entrance exams out there including the Health Education Systems Inc. (HESI), Test of Essential Academic Skills (TEAS), Nursing Entrance Test (NET), and Health Occupations Basic Entrance Test (HOBET).

Starting your career off on the right foot can make all the difference, and your nursing entrance exam scores can be the key to admission into the nursing school of your choice. It is also a good indicator of your chances for success in a nursing program of study. Additionally, many people who are already in nursing school may need to take the test again either while pursuing a degree or as a precursor to the NCLEX examination.

Find out which exam your future school requires and look for resources to study for that exam. There are tons of test preparation books and practice questions available for you. Another good idea may be to ask someone who went through your target program and ask what they used to study for the examinations.

7 TIME TO BECOME A NURSE!

What exactly does it mean to become a nurse? There are a two types of nurses, they are Licensed Practical Nurse (LPN) and Registered Nurse (RN). To make things more confusing, there are a few different programs you can do to become an RN that result in different degrees. Yes, that sounds complex, but don't fret. I will spell it out for you.

Let's begin with Licensed Practical Nurse (LPN). LPN's are nurses who care for patients under the direction of a Registered Nurse (RN). LPN's earn a practical nursing degree, typically in 12-36 months, and can be placed in the workforce much sooner than RNs. The LPN license has a few stipulations, which can vary state to state. The list may include not being able to initiate or mange intravenous (IV) lines, not being able to administer certain medications, and the delegation of some tasks to another nursing staff. In addition, career advancement could be limited.

Despite this, becoming an LPN is still an attractive option. Upon completion of the LPN program, you will need to sit for the national licensure exam called NCLEX-PN. The job outlook is very bright for LPN's. As an LPN, you have numerous opportunities from Skilled Nursing and Rehabilitation Facilities to Long Term Care Facilities, Occupational Health jobs, physicians' offices, administrative jobs, or even outpatient offices. You may ask, "What about hospitals?" The answer is many of the larger hospitals have a nursing workforce comprised mainly of RNs.

Please do not let that deter you. As stated before, becoming an LPN is the quickest way to get out into the world and begin working as a nurse. Licensed practical nursing could be a good choice because many RN programs have bridge options available for LPNs. This will allow you to continue working while studying to become a registered nurse. Let us look closer at the web of nursing.

8 BECOMING A REGISTERED NURSE (ADN)

There are two different educational structures that lead you to become an RN. The first is Associate Degree in Nursing (ADN). This program is usually shorter in duration than Bachelors of Science in Nursing (BSN). ADN programs are often offered at community colleges and some universities. They typically last from two to three years. After completing an ADN program, you will have an Associate's Degree and be able to sit for the NCLEX-RN.

You may ask why ADN program over LPN if they are similar in length? Well, the answer depends on your needs. If you are planning to earn a higher degree in the future, ADN may be a good starting point for you. However, if you would like to begin working as a nurse as quickly as possible, LPN may be a better option. Should you decide to go after the ADN program immediately, you will have all the basics covered for the BSN and will only need some additional courses to attain a Bachelors in Nursing in the future. If you do a quick search on Nursing programs, you should be able to find one that will fit your needs.

9 BACHELORS OF SCIENCE IN NURSE (BSN)

The other educational structure is obtaining a BSN or Bachelors of Science in Nursing. This is a 4-year degree that is widely offered throughout the country. It also will require you sit for the NCLEX-RN. There are a ton of BSN programs many of which offer non-traditional routes to attain the BSN. Here are a few examples: LPN to BSN bridge program, Accelerated BSN program, and RN to BSN program.

Let me elaborate on the programs listed above. LPN to BSN is a shortened program for licensed practical nurses to take that includes all the courses to attain the degree as well as a few clinical hours that may be needed. Most programs like this are structured in a way that is feasible for someone already working as a nurse. They may offer evening or weekend programs.

Accelerated BSN programs are for people who already hold a bachelor's degree in an area other than nursing. This is the route I took to nursing. You enroll in the program after making sure you have all the prerequisites for the nursing program. After you have been accepted to the program, you will take only nursing lectures and clinical courses. The accelerated programs typically last between 12 to 18 months, averaging about 15 months. Following the completion, you will be able to sit for the NCLEX-RN examination.

Lastly, RN to BSN programs are for those people who went through the ADN programs and are now completing only the bachelor portion. These people have already sat for the NCLEX-RN and may already be working as RNs. These programs were designed to be completed in about one year and are composed of the remaining courses that were not taken during the ADN program, which often includes research and statistics classes. There are many different offerings for these programs and often can be completed online, to allow you to continue working while taking classes.

Bonus two cents

I would like to share some personal advice with you. Choose the route that makes more sense for your life. As you can see, all roads lead to nursing; however, there are some advantages to different routes. If you have the time and ability to get a 4-year degree, I strongly encourage you to do it.

I have been looking at how the field is evolving and changing for the better. There are certain requirements that will likely come up in the next several years. There is a push for all nurses to attain bachelor degrees. It is being made easier for those who are already RNs, and some jobs' benefits include help with paying for school. It makes sense to consider the BSN option.

Also, some hospital systems are going after a prestigious recognition called Magnet. Magnet Recognition means the hospital has attained the highest standards among healthcare organizations. The Magnet Recognition is only attained by a small percentage of healthcare systems in the United States. Magnet mean the hospital is committed to nursing excellence and top-notch patient care. Some facilities with Magnet distinction are required to have a certain percentage of RNs holding a BSN degree, performing a certain amount of research, and continuing to advance the field of nursing. Magnet facilities have also been shown to be great places to work for nurses and to employ nurses that are more satisfied with their jobs. There also are often career ladders that allow you to advance within clinical nursing without going back to school.

One more tip, the last semester of nursing school you will likely be completing a preceptorship which is an internship for student nurses that are in the very last semester of nursing school. My advice is to start working a few semesters ahead of time to try to get on a unit that is of interest to you. For example, if you are interested in cardiac nursing, try to get time on a cardiac unit. The purpose of that last semester is to get some experience training one on one before attaining your first job. Choose wisely.

10 WILL IT BE EASY?

My answer to the question above is a very confident no! Nothing about nursing school will be easy, but it will be well worth it. You will go through every emotion known to man. You will think "this is crazy," "this is a bad idea," or "I am just going to quit." My advice is don't quit; don't give up; and just keep going.

Ask any nurses you meet and they will tell you the process was hard, but it is one of the best decisions they ever made. If you get into nursing for the right reasons, you will begin to realize the how much of an impact you can have on people's lives.

The key to making it is finding the appropriate school/life or school/work/life balance. Most nursing students lose all grips on life balance. Do not get it wrong; nursing school is demanding. If you do not take the time to unwind, you will have a very stressful time.

Organization is critical

It will be extremely important for you to be organized. Depending on which program you choose, the courses may move quickly. Organization will be the key to staying on task. Figure out what will keep you organized. Do you do well with paper planners? Are you a digital calendar kind of person? What about Task/To-Do lists? Maybe you will use them all. No matter which you choose, decide early and stay on top of your organization from the very beginning.

Schedules make life easier

The second tip is to schedule everything. This goes from study time to downtime, to family and friend time. Schedule as far in advance as you can and stick to the plan. No one likes to make plans to hang out with you and get cancelled on at the last minute. Do not become the "I am just too busy" person. You will be busy, but you need to remain sane throughout the process. Scheduling your time can help keep you sane.

Communication keeps relationships healthy

Last, but not least, let your friends and family know you will need their help. Be up front with them. Make sure they know you will be occupied at times, but you are committed to keeping the plans with them and not missing out on every important thing that goes on. By that same token, let them know you may not be able to attend every event. But you will do your best to attend the things you can. You will also need their moral and emotional support. This can be a rollercoaster for everyone, but it does not have to be the worse ride ever.

Ask for help and delegate tasks

One thing you will learn in nursing school is to delegate. Delegation and teamwork are foundations in nursing that are very useful in your personal life as well. You may need to delegate some things that were previously your responsibility. While every nurse thinks of him/herself as super human, there are still times when we need help too. Do not be afraid to ask. Surely your family and friends are willing to go that extra mile for you.

11 WHEW, YOU MADE IT!

You have arrived at graduation! See, I told you you'd make it. Congratulations on getting to the end of your nursing program. Again, you have made it through a very important milestone. Now it is time to decide where you want to kick start your career. After graduation, you will be focusing on passing the NCLEX examination. We will discuss the exam later. Let's celebrate your accomplishment!

Graduating from nursing school often includes a "Pinning" ceremony, which is a tradition in the profession. The Pinning ceremony is symbolic of welcoming the new graduate into the profession. Often the ceremony is around graduation and the new nurses are presented with a pin by nursing faculty or a special person in your life. It is an exciting time and a major stepping stone.

er graduation and pinning have taken place, check on your transcript. Your state's board g will request the final copy of the transcript. After graduation, you may feel confused. Most likely, no one spelled out the steps that needed to be taken to move into your career, which can make the process longer and more drawn out.

Again, do not fret. Here is what you need to do. Grab a pen and create a list. Here is a sample To-Do List you may want to consider for graduation and immediately following.

To- Do:

- Submit your transcript request so the school can send your transcript to your designated Board of Nursing (money may be required)

- Register or find a review for the NCLEX (money may be required)

- Apply to take the NCLEX (money required)

- Create a study schedule

- After receiving your Authorization to Test (ATT), register and choose a NCLEX test date

- Begin a preliminary job search

- Update your resume

- Make a list of job wants and needs

- Do your research when it comes to income wants/needs

- Consider joining a professional nursing organization

This is a good starting point for you to be organized and transition as easily and quickly as possible. There will be a time period directly after graduation when the Board of Nursing will need to process all the applications to test that it received. Depending on the time of year you graduate, the process could take longer. May is a very common graduation time. Therefore, it takes longer to get an authorization to test. August or Fall graduation is the second most popular, and lastly December. Keep this in mind when planning and studying. Try to keep your stress about this process, which you have little control over, as low as possible.

Each state has specific criteria you must meet to become licensed as a nurse. Here is a compiled list of all 50 states and the District of Columbia's Boards of Nursing. Please visit your state Board of Nursing's website to find out exactly what you will need for licensure.

Alabama
www.abn.alabama.gov

Alaska
www.commerce.alaska.gov

Arizona
www.azbn.gov

Arkansas
www.arsbn.arkansas.gov

California
www.rn.ca.gov

Colorado
www.colorado.gov/pacific/dora/Nursing

Connecticut
www.ct.gov/dph/cwp

Delaware
www.dpr.deleware.gov/boards/nursing/

Florida
www.floridanursing.gov

Georgia
www.sos.ga.gov/index.php/licensing/plb/45

Hawaii
www.cca.hawaii.gov/pvl/boards/nursing/

Idaho
www.ibn.idaho.gov/

Illinois
www.idfpr.com/profs/Nursing.asp

Indiana
www.in.gov/pla/nursing.htm

Iowa
www.nursing.iowa.gov

Kansas
www.ksbn.org

Kentucky
www.kbn.ky.gov

Louisiana
www.lsbn.state.la.us

Maine
www.maine.gov/boardofnursing/

Maryland
www.mbon.maryland.gov/

Massachusetts
www.mass.gov/eohhs/gov/departments/dph/progra
ms/hcq/dhpl/nursing

Michigan
www.michigan.gov/

Minnesota
www.mn.gov/boards/nursing/

Mississippi
www.msbn.ms.gov

Missouri
www.pr.mo.gov/nursing.asp

Montana
www.nurse.mt.gov

Nebraska
www.dhhs.ne.gov/publichealth/Pages/crl_nursing_nu
rsingindex.aspx

Nevada
www.nevadanursingboard.org

New Hampshire
www.nh.gov/nursing/

New Jersey
www.njconsumeraffairs.gov/nur/Pages/default.aspx

New Mexico
www.nmbon.sks.com

New York
www.op.nysed.gov/prof/nurse

North Carolina
www.ncbon.com

North Dakota
www.ndbon.org/

Ohio
www.nursing.ohio.gov/

Oklahoma
www.nursing.ok.gov/

Oregon
www.oregan.gov/OSBN/pages/rn-lpnlicensure.aspx

Pennsylvania
www.dos.pa.gov/nurse

Rhode Island
www.health.ri.gov/nursing

South Carolina
www.llr.state.sc.us/pol/nursing/

South Dakota
www.doh.sd.gov/boards/nursing

Tennessee
www.tn.gov/health/topic/nursing-board

Texas
www.bon.texas.gov/

Utah
www.dopl.utah.gov/licensing/nursing.html

Vermont
www.sec.state.vt.us

Virginia
www.dhp.virginia.gov/nursing/

Washington
www.doh.wa.gov/LicensesPermitsandCertificates/Nur
singCommission

Washington DC
www.doh.dc.gov/service/board-nursing

West Virginia
www.wvrnboard.com

Wisconsin
www.psps.wi.gov/Default.aspx

Wyoming
www.nursing-online.state.wy.us

12 NCLEX TIME!

This is the moment you have been working so hard for. All the blood, sweat, and tears culminate here. For a lot of you, this is the most important test you will ever take. I suggested earlier that you take a review course for the test. If you do not have the ability to take one, you still must dedicate plenty of time to studying. Study. Study harder. Then, study some more.

There are millions of test preparation resources for the NCLEX. The purpose of this book is not to teach you how to pass the examination; however, here are a few tips that worked for me or that I have gathered from other nurses. First, do a review of the nursing process. Be familiar with age-specific considerations for nursing, for example, the developmental milestones of a preschooler and special considerations for administering medication to the elderly.

The NCLEX is largely based on safety. In fact, the purpose of the test is to help insure you will practice nursing safely and not knowingly do harm to those you are caring for. Study with safety in mind. Do as many practice questions as you can after you have reviewed. You will the get to see how the questions are formulated and how to think through answering the questions.

The NCLEX examination is an adaptive test. This means the test adapts the questions based on your strengths and weakness of answering. There is a test bank which includes some questions that will not contribute to your score, but possibly will be used on future exams. The test will end once you have reached a certain percentage of questions answered correctly or incorrectly.

At the time of this book was written, the NCLEX examination fee was about $200.00 for nurses seeking licensure in the United States. The National Council of State Boards of Nursing (www.ncsbn.org) has all the information you will need regarding the NCLEX. You will register for the test on the NCSBN site. Plans of actions for before the test, examination day, and after testing can be found there. The NCSBN suggests you download and read the most current Test

Plan as you are preparing for the examination. The Test Plan lays out the categories that will are included in the test and can help focus your studies.

Be as prepared as you can before testing, and you will be fine. If you were able to make it through nursing school, you can pass this examination. Remain calm, breathe, and answer the questions as logically as you can. You've got this!

After taking the examination, you will receive your results. You must make sure your designated Board of Nursing receive them so your nursing license can be processed. It will be posted on the website for verification purposes. You will need your examination pass date or actual licensure date. After these things take place, you are official.

13 STARTING YOUR JOB SEARCH

After you have passed the NCLEX, you will feel a tremendous amount of relief. Then, the daunting task of finding a job begins. There are several websites that will be helpful in your jobs search. First, you will need to make sure your resume is in tip-top shape. Your resume will either get you in the door or turned away. Spend time and energy on your resume. It is an important representation of you. Below is a chart comparing the average salary in the United States to the average registered nurse salary.

	Hourly Wage	Weekly Wage	Monthly Salary	Annual Salary
Registered Nurse Average Salary	$32.66	$1,306	$5,660	$67,930
U.S. National Average Salary	$22.01	$880	$3,815	$45,790

http://nursesalaryguide.net/registered-nurse-rn-salary/

Many schools have career centers that may have relationships with facilities and job posting. I recommend you start there. Networking can also play a big part in finding your ideal job. Use your connections to your advantage. Join social media networks. Develop a profile on LinkedIn; many companies recruit through this site. A few other popular sites are:

> www.healthcareers.com
> www.indeed.com
> www.nursingjobs.com

All of these are good starting points for career searching. It is also a good idea to apply to the local hospitals in your area.

After applying for jobs, it is a good time to sharpen your interviewing skills. Think about how you would answer questions asking about your strengths and weaknesses. Interview questions often ask how you plan to handle a particularly challenging issue. Be ready to answer. Practice. Have friends and family help you by holding mock interviews. This way you will not be surprised or put on the spot by any of the questions. Confidence is key to getting the job! Proper preparation will never steer you wrong. Good luck on securing your first nursing job. You will be as awesome as you proclaimed you would be when this journey first started.

Myth: All new nurses must start on a medical surgical unit.

Fact: NOT TRUE. It is true medical surgical nurses are well rounded; however, it would also benefit you to start in a place you desire, and that can nurture your growth in the profession.

14 A DAY IN THE LIFE OF A NURSE

A majority of nurses work in a hospital setting; therefore, this description will be from the hospital perspective. Twelve-hour shifts are the most common work schedule. Typically, you arrive 30 to 40 minutes before the shift will start. That is because you need to mentally prepare for the shift. Most likely, you will have three to six patients you are responsible for. You will get a report from the previous nurse on the specific medical history, reason for hospitalization, interventions to be carried out, and medications. After you have finished getting the report on your patients, you will have a brief moment to get more pertinent information from the individual patient charts.

Now, it is time to prioritize your to-do list for the shift. You may need to start passing out medication at this time. If not, you may go see each patient and introduce yourself. You may also have time to do head-to-toe assessments on the patients. Other nurses may choose to do the assessments while giving the medications. There is no right or wrong way. In addition to medications, there could be a host of other things needed by each patient. For example, you may need to draw blood, collect specimens, change wound dressings, feed, and even adjust immobile patients.

These activities take place throughout the shift and may need to be done around the same time or spread out. You have the power to decide how your day will be set up. If you are lucky, you will have a CNA working with you to assist with the things you need to do during the shift. There are times when patients are demanding and require a lot of your time. You will need to be able to manage your time efficiently and effectively.

There will be days when you run around so much you do not even have time to use the restroom. If you get a break, cherish it. The physicians will come around and may change the orders, interventions, or medications. You are responsible for being updated at all times during the shift. You have a short amount of time to build rapport and positively impact someone's life. Helping and giving are a part of your daily life. At the end of the shift, you will need to make sure all your ducks are in a row before the next shift of nurses arrive. When the next nurse arrives, you will need to give her a report and update her on everything that happened on your shift. As long as you have accurately documented everything you did during your shift, you can go home. That was a small glimpse into the day in the life of a nurse.

Story Time

There have been moments during my career that have made me question my decision to become a nurse, especially experiencing loss repeatedly. When that happens, I like to think about some of the happy occasions that I have experienced. Those thoughts help me remember why I do this. I would like to share a story with you.

I was working on a pediatric cardiac unit. In that unit, we cared for children that were born with various heart conditions, some even deemed as fatal. There was a resilient little baby that was having a hard time recovering from one of the many cardiac surgeries he had undergone. The last surgery did not go so well. He had a few cardiac arrests. The nurses spent as much time as possible snuggling him, holding him, and just sitting in his hospital room with him, night in and night out. Eventually, he was able to go home. As time flew by, we wondered how he was doing out in the real world. One morning, to our surprise he came walking on the unit. He looked amazing! He was healthy and thriving. He was about two-years-old at the time. We hugged and kissed him as if he was our very own child. In that moment, I knew I was doing the work I was created to do.

15 CONCLUSION

On behalf of the over 3.9 million active nurses in the United States of America, I would like to welcome you to the wonderful world of nursing. We are so glad you decided to join us. We wish you a lifetime of happiness and fulfillment from the profession. I pray you dedicate your life to healing the sick, nurturing people back to health, and loving every minute of it. I hope you positively touch every life that comes into contact with you. This is only the beginning. You will have plenty of time and opportunity to spread your wings. Good luck. I know you will be a great nurse!

"For the sick, it is important to have the best." –
Florence Nightingale

RESOURCE LIST

Visit www.couchtocareer.com for more information and Career Coaching services.

www.allnuringschools.com - "Certified Nursing Assistant Overview." Certified Nursing Assistant Quick Facts. N.p., n.d. Web. 30 Aug. 2016.

www.allnursingschools.com - CNA Salary and Job Growth." Certified Nursing Assistant Salary. N.p., n.d. Web. 30 Aug. 2016.

www.nursingassistants.net -"Everything You Want To Know About Being A CNA." Nursing Assistant Resources On the Web RSS. N.p., n.d. Web. 30 Aug. 2016.

www.mycnajobs.com/caregiver-cna-pay/ - Experience , By. "Caregiver, HHA, & CNA Pay." CNA, Caregiver, and HHA Jobs. N.p., n.d. Web. 30 Aug. 2016.

www.healthcareers.com

www.indeed.com

www.nursingjobs.com

http://nursesalaryguide.net/registered-nurse-rn-salary/ - "Registered Nurse RN Salary - Nurse Salary Guide." Nurse Salary Guide. N.p., n.d. Web. 30 Aug. 2016